How to Get Wet for Sex

25+ Hot and Slippery Ways to Increase Vaginal Lubrication, Get Aroused Really Fast, and Break Your Dry Spell plus Tips to Solve Vaginal Dryness and Overcome Painful Intercourse

Cheryl Bach

How to Get Wet for Sex

Cheryl Bach

Table of Contents

Chapter I.

Introduction

A. Why Vaginal Lubrication Is Important for Sexual Pleasure and Overall Sexual Health

Sexual pleasure is an essential component of one's emotional and physical well-being, and vaginal lubrication is a critical aspect of sexual pleasure. The vaginal lubrication facilitates smooth penetration and reduces discomfort or pain during sexual intercourse. Lubrication aids in reducing vaginal tears or injuries during penetration which can increase the risk of infections and sexually transmitted infections.

Additionally, vaginal lubrication can make sex enjoyable while increasing the level of pleasure. Vaginal lubrication is necessary to maintain a healthy pH balance and prevent dryness of the vaginal tissues and the vulva which helps keep your vulva and vagina healthy.

B. Common Causes of Vaginal Dryness and Painful Intercourse

There are several factors that can cause vaginal dryness leading to painful intercourse. Hormonal changes due to menstruation, pregnancy, breastfeeding, menopause and medical conditions like Sjogren's syndrome, an autoimmune disease that affects the body's moisture-producing glands, and lichen sclerosus, a skin condition that can cause itching, burning and scarring around the vulva and vaginal opening can cause vaginal dryness.

Certain medications used to treat depression, allergies and hypertension as well as smoking, excessive alcohol intake and poor nutrition habits are also factors that can contribute to vaginal dryness.

Painful sexual intercourse, also known as dyspareunia, can be caused by vaginal infections such as yeast infections, bacterial vaginosis, or sexually transmitted infections. Other factors that can cause painful intercourse include vulvodynia, a chronic pain disorder affecting the vulva, or vaginismus, a condition where muscles in the vagina involuntarily tighten during penetration.

C. The Goal of the Book

The goal of the book is to provide practical and effective ways to increase vaginal lubrication, arousal, and pleasure.

The purpose of this book is to offer practical and effective solutions to women who experience vaginal dryness, painful intercourse, or those who seek to enhance their sexual pleasure. This book provides 25+ hot and slippery ways to increase vaginal lubrication, get aroused really fast, and break your dry spell.

How to Get Wet for Sex

You will learn how to identify the factors that cause vaginal dryness, and how to overcome them. There are various treatments, such as using certain types of lubes, natural remedies, hormonal therapies, and lifestyle changes that can help increase lubrication, improve arousal, and make sex more pleasurable.

This book aims to help you discover the paths to sexual satisfaction by providing you with useful information, practical advice, and different approaches to enhance your sexual experience. In addition, this book also provides tips on how to solve vaginal dryness, and overcome painful intercourse so that you can enjoy a fulfilling sex life.

Whether you are a young woman who experiences occasional vaginal dryness or a menopausal woman struggling with persistent symptoms, this book has insights, recommendations, and solutions that will benefit you. The primary goal of this book is to empower women with the knowledge and tools they need to optimize their sexual health, increase their pleasure, and overall well-being.

Through reading this book, you will gain a deeper understanding of the importance of vaginal lubrication, and how it impacts sexual pleasure, health, and relationships. You will also learn practical ways to overcome vaginal dryness, plus tips to enhance your sexual experience and make sex more enjoyable and fulfilling.

So sit back, relax, and get ready to discover a whole new world of sexual pleasure and satisfaction. Whether you want to spice up your sex life or improve your overall sexual health, this book is a valuable resource that offers guidance, insights, and tips to help you achieve your sexual goals.

By following the recommendations outlined in this book, you can overcome the challenges associated with vaginal dryness or painful intercourse, and achieve a fulfilling sex life. So why wait? Let's dive in and explore the countless ways to increase your lubrication, boost your arousal, and get that slippery, hot, and steamy sexual experience that you've been dreaming of!

Chapter II.

Understanding Vaginal Lubrication

A. Overview of the Anatomy and Physiology of Vaginal Lubrication

To understand vaginal lubrication, it is necessary to have a basic understanding of the female reproductive system's anatomy and physiology. The vulva is the outer part of the female genitalia, which includes the labia, clitoris, urethra, and vaginal opening. The vagina sits behind the vulva and is a muscular canal that connects the uterus to the outside of the body.

Vaginal lubrication happens via two glands. There is the Skene's gland which is adjacent to the urethra and the Bartholin's gland which is located on either side of the lower end of the vaginal opening. These glands produce and release fluid in response to arousal.

During sexual arousal, the blood flow to the genital area increases, causing the glands to produce more fluid. This fluid is then released through the vaginal opening, providing lubrication for sexual intercourse. The amount of lubrication produced can vary depending on factors such as age, hormones, and level of arousal, which will be discussed in more detail later in this chapter.

B. Types of Lubrication and How They Vary with Age, Hormones, and Arousal Level

There are two main types of vaginal lubrication: natural and artificial. Natural lubrication is the kind produced by the body during sexual arousal, while artificial lubrication is added externally using various lubricants such as water-based, silicone-based, or oil-based lubes.

As women age, the amount of natural lubrication produced by the body tends to decrease due to a decrease in hormones. During menopause, the reduction in estrogen levels can lead to significant vaginal dryness, making sex painful or uncomfortable.

Hormones also play a significant role in vaginal lubrication, as estrogen is essential for maintaining the thickness and elasticity of the vaginal walls. Hormonal changes during the menstrual cycle can also affect the amount and consistency of natural lubrication.

Arousal level also affects vaginal lubrication. Women who are highly aroused tend to produce more natural lubrication than those who are not as aroused. Stress and anxiety can also inhibit natural lubrication production, leading to vaginal dryness.

C. Effects of Stress, Medications, Menopause, and Other Factors on Vaginal Lubrication

Stress can have a significant impact on vaginal lubrication. When the body is under stress, it releases cortisol, a hormone that can inhibit arousal and reduce lubrication production. Additionally, medications such as antidepressants, antihistamines, and some birth control pills can cause vaginal dryness as a side effect of their actions on hormone levels and blood flow to the genital area.

Menopause is also a significant factor that impacts vaginal lubrication. As estrogen levels decrease, the vaginal walls can become thin and dry. This can result in pain or discomfort during sexual intercourse. Women undergoing menopause may also experience hot flashes, night sweats, and vaginal itching, which can further exacerbate dryness.

Other factors that can impact vaginal lubrication include breastfeeding, certain medical conditions such as cancer treatments, and radiation therapy. These treatments can affect the body's hormone levels and reduce blood flow to the genital area, leading to vaginal dryness.

In summary, understanding vaginal lubrication is essential to achieving sexual pleasure and maintaining good sexual health. While some factors like age and menopause cannot be prevented, there are various methods and strategies for increasing lubrication and overcoming vaginal dryness. In the next chapter, we will explore 25+ hot and slippery ways to increase vaginal lubrication, get aroused quickly, and overcome dry spells. With these tips, women can enhance their sexual pleasure, boost their intimacy, and improve their overall sexual health.

How to Get Wet for Sex

Chapter III.

25+ Hot and Slippery Ways to Increase Vaginal Lubrication and Arousal

In this chapter, we will discuss 25+ hot and slippery ways to increase vaginal lubrication and arousal. These techniques are designed to help women overcome dry spells, boost their sexual pleasure, and improve their overall sexual health.

A. Psychological Techniques

Eliminating Stress and Anxiety: Stress and anxiety can inhibit natural lubrication production. To combat this, it's essential to try and eliminate stress and anxiety as much as possible. Some techniques that can help include deep breathing, exercise, and engaging in enjoyable activities.

Incorporating Relaxation Techniques like Meditation or Mindfulness: Meditation and mindfulness can help decrease stress and anxiety and increase relaxation. It can also increase body awareness that allows you to better understand what works for your body and what doesn't. Take a few minutes each day to meditate or practice mindfulness, focusing on deep breathing and relaxation.

Boosting Confidence: Confidence is key when it comes to sexual pleasure. Embrace your sexuality and own your desires and preferences. You can boost your confidence by practicing positive affirmations, self-care, and surrounding yourself with supportive people who encourage your sexual exploration.

B. Physical Techniques

Foreplay and Sensual Touch: Foreplay and sensual touch can help increase blood flow to the genital area and promote vaginal lubrication. Engage in teasing, kissing, and caressing to increase arousal before initiating intercourse.

Incorporating Sex Toys like Vibrators or Lubricants: Sex toys can help increase pleasure and stimulate lubrication production. Vibrators can increase arousal and provide clitoral stimulation, while lubricants can enhance sensation and reduce friction during sex. Experiment with different lubricants or sex toys and see what works best for you. Water-based lubricants are safe to use with condoms, while silicone-based lubricants are long-lasting.

Different Positions that Can Help Increase Stimulation: Different sexual positions can help increase stimulation and promote vaginal lubrication. For example, being on top can allow you to control the pace and angles of penetration, increasing clitoral stimulation and promoting natural lubrication.

Health Tips that Can Contribute to a Healthier Vagina: A healthy vagina is more likely to produce adequate natural lubrication. Practice good hygiene by washing the genital area daily with mild soap and water. Wear cotton underwear and avoid tight clothing that can trap moisture and lead to infections. Stay hydrated and eat a healthy diet rich in probiotics, which can support vaginal health.

Understanding the Role of Using Condoms: Using condoms can help prevent the transmission of sexually transmitted infections and unintended pregnancies. However, condoms can also contribute to vaginal dryness. To combat this, try adding a drop of water-based lubricant inside the condom before use. This can enhance sensation and reduce friction, promoting natural lubrication.

Cheryl Bach

Kegel Exercises: Kegel exercises can help strengthen the pelvic floor muscles and promote blood flow to the genital area. Strong pelvic floor muscles can lead to increased sensitivity and more intense orgasms. To perform Kegel exercises, contract and hold the muscles used to stop urine flow for several seconds and then release.

Nipple Play: Nipple play can help increase blood flow to the genital area and promote arousal and vaginal lubrication. Try gentle sucking or caressing of the nipples during foreplay.

Role-Playing: Role-playing can be a fun and exciting way to spice up your sex life. Embodying different characters can help increase arousal and promote natural lubrication. Talk with your partner about your fantasies and experiment with role-playing scenarios.

How to Get Wet for Sex

Dirty Talk: Dirty talk can be a powerful tool for getting aroused and promoting vaginal lubrication. Communicate your desires and fantasies to your partner, using explicit language to heighten anticipation and arousal.

Sensory Play: Sensory play involving the use of textures, scents, and tastes can help increase arousal and promote natural lubrication. Experiment with different textures such as silk or velvet, and try incorporating scents like sandalwood or jasmine into your lovemaking.

Lubricants: Lubricants can enhance sensation and reduce friction, promoting natural lubrication. Experiment with different types of lubricants, such as water-based or silicone-based, to find one that works best for you. Be sure to choose a lubricant that is safe to use with condoms and other sex toys.

Cheryl Bach

Slow and Steady: Taking things slow and steady can help increase arousal and promote natural lubrication. Focus on exploring each other's bodies, using gentle touches and kisses to build anticipation and desire.

Shower Sex: Shower sex can be a great way to increase stimulation, promote relaxation, and enhance natural lubrication. The warm water can help relax the body and promote blood flow to the genital area, making sex more enjoyable.

Erotic Massage: An erotic massage can help increase arousal and promote natural lubrication. Use light pressure and long, slow strokes to stimulate erogenous zones such as the neck, ears, nipples, and inner thighs.

Experiment with Temperature Play: Temperature play involving the use of hot and cold sensations can help increase arousal and promote natural lubrication. Try placing a warm towel over your genital area or using ice cubes to stimulate the nipples and genitals during foreplay.

Communication: The most important factor in promoting natural lubrication is communication with your partner. Talk openly about what feels good and what doesn't, and be open to exploration and experimentation. Trust your body and your instincts, and allow yourself to fully embrace your desires and passions.

Chapter IV.

Tips to Overcome Painful Intercourse and Vaginal Dryness

Sex should be a pleasurable experience for all parties involved. Unfortunately, many women suffer from painful intercourse or vaginal dryness, which can make sex uncomfortable or even unbearable. If you are experiencing these issues, it's essential to talk to your doctor to rule out any underlying medical conditions. Below are some tips that can help you overcome painful intercourse and vaginal dryness.

A. Overview of What Causes Painful Sex and How to Manage Associated Issues

Painful intercourse can be caused by various factors, including hormonal changes, infections, vaginal dryness, lack of lubrication, and psychological issues such as stress and anxiety. To manage associated issues, it is crucial to get an accurate diagnosis and treatment plan from your healthcare provider. Depending on the underlying cause, treatment may involve medication, surgery, or lifestyle changes. Psychological therapy can also be beneficial in addressing anxiety or trauma-related issues that may be contributing to painful intercourse.

B. Lubrication Options and How to Choose the Right Lube

One of the most effective ways to combat vaginal dryness is to use a lubricant during sex. There are many different types of lubricants available, including water-based, silicone-based, and oil-based options. It's important to choose the right lube for your body and your needs, as some types may be more irritating than others. For example, oil-based lubes can break down latex condoms and increase the risk of STI transmission.

When choosing a lubricant, consider factors such as the ingredients, consistency, and intended use. Water-based lubes are safe to use with condoms and can be easily washed off, while silicone-based lubes last longer and feel more slippery. Hybrid lubes are a combination of both water and silicone-based, offering both the benefits of longer-lasting lubrication and easier clean-up.

It's also important to consider any sensitivities or allergies that you may have when choosing a lube. Some people may be allergic to certain ingredients, such as glycerin or propylene glycol, which can cause irritation or discomfort. To avoid this, look for lubes that are free from these ingredients or opt for natural, organic products.

C. Natural Remedies

Herbal Supplements or Teas: Certain herbs and supplements have been shown to improve vaginal lubrication and reduce painful intercourse. For example, evening primrose oil contains omega-6 fatty acids that can help reduce inflammation and boost natural lubrication. Black cohosh has also been shown to have estrogen-like effects, which can help reduce vaginal dryness.

Other herbs and supplements that may improve vaginal health include dong quai, ginseng, red clover, and chaste tree berry. However, it's important to talk to your healthcare provider before taking any supplements or herbal remedies, as they can interact with medications or have side effects.

Avoiding Common Irritants: Certain products can cause irritation or dryness in the genital area, which can contribute to painful intercourse and vaginal dryness. These products

Cheryl Bach

include harsh soaps, douches, scented tampons, and some types of underwear.

To avoid irritation, use mild, unscented soaps and avoid using douches or other cleansing products inside the vagina. Opt for cotton underwear and avoid tight-fitting clothes that can cause sweating and irritation.

Lifestyle Changes that Can Help Combat Vaginal Dryness: Lifestyle changes can also play a role in improving vaginal health and reducing painful intercourse. For example, staying hydrated by drinking plenty of water throughout the day can help keep the body moisturized and reduce dryness. Eating a balanced diet that includes plenty of fruits, vegetables, and healthy fats can also help improve overall vaginal health.

Regular exercise can also help improve blood flow to the genitals and boost natural lubrication. Kegel exercises, which involve squeezing and releasing the muscles in the pelvic floor, can help strengthen these muscles and improve overall vaginal health.

D. Medical Treatments

In some cases, medical treatments may be necessary to address painful intercourse and vaginal dryness. Your healthcare provider can recommend the best options based on your specific needs and concerns.

Medication: There are several medications that can help improve vaginal dryness and reduce painful intercourse. Hormone replacement therapy, which involves taking estrogen and/or progesterone to replace declining hormone levels, can help improve natural lubrication and reduce discomfort.

Topical moisturizers and lubricants can also be used to improve lubrication and reduce discomfort during intercourse. Some medications, such as antidepressants and antihistamines, can cause vaginal dryness as a side effect. If you are experiencing vaginal dryness as a side effect of medication, your healthcare provider may be able to adjust your medication or recommend alternatives.

Surgery: In rare cases, surgery may be necessary to address painful intercourse or vaginal dryness. Procedures such as vaginoplasty or labiaplasty can be used to address structural issues or improve overall vaginal health.

However, it's important to note that surgery is not always necessary and should only be considered as a last resort option. Your healthcare provider will discuss all available options with you and help you determine the best course of treatment based on your specific needs and concerns.

How to Get Wet for Sex

In conclusion, painful intercourse and vaginal dryness can be frustrating and uncomfortable, but there are many options available to improve vaginal health and reduce discomfort. From natural remedies to medical treatments, there are many ways to overcome these issues and enjoy a fulfilling sex life with your partner. It's important to talk to your healthcare provider about any concerns you may have and to explore all available options together.

Remember, there is no one-size-fits-all solution when it comes to vaginal health and sexual wellness. What works for one person may not work for another, so it's important to explore different options and find what works best for you.

By taking steps to improve your vaginal health and reduce painful intercourse, you can not only enjoy a more comfortable sex life but also improve your overall quality of life. Don't be afraid to seek help and explore different options – you deserve to feel comfortable and confident in your own body.

Chapter V.

Understanding your Sexual Health

A. Importance of Regular Gynecological Appointments

Regular gynecological appointments are an essential part of taking care of your sexual health. During these appointments, your healthcare provider will perform a physical exam and a Pap smear to screen for cervical cancer. They may also perform a breast exam and a pelvic exam to check for any abnormalities or signs of infection.

It's important to see your healthcare provider at least once a year for a gynecological exam, even if you are not sexually active. This allows for early detection and treatment of any potential issues, and can help keep you healthy and sexually empowered.

Cheryl Bach

B. Tracking Your Menstrual Cycle

Keeping track of your menstrual cycle can also be an important part of understanding your sexual health. By tracking your menstrual cycle, you can better predict when you are most fertile and plan for safe sex. It can also alert you to any changes or irregularities in your cycle that may indicate an underlying issue, such as hormonal imbalances or pregnancy.

There are several ways to track your menstrual cycle, including using a calendar or app to record the start and end of your period each month. You can also track changes in cervical mucus and basal body temperature to determine when ovulation is occurring.

By understanding your menstrual cycle, you can make informed decisions about contraception and family planning. It's also important to discuss any concerns or irregularities with your healthcare provider.

C. Communicating Your Needs and Concerns with Your Partner

Open and honest communication is essential for a healthy and fulfilling sexual relationship. It's important to talk to your partner about your needs and concerns, including any issues with lubrication or pain during intercourse.

Your partner should be supportive and willing to work with you to find solutions to any sexual health issues you may be experiencing. This may include exploring different positions or using lubricants to help with vaginal dryness.

It's also important to discuss and practice safe sex, including the use of contraceptives and regular testing for sexually transmitted infections (STIs).

If you are experiencing painful intercourse or other sexual health issues, it's important to seek medical attention and speak openly with your healthcare provider about any concerns or questions you may have.

Additionally, it's important to remember that everyone's experience with sexual health is unique, and there is no right or wrong way to feel or experience things. By prioritizing open communication and seeking out resources and support when needed, you can take control of your sexual health and enjoy a happy and fulfilling sex life.

Chapter VI.

Conclusion

Congratulations on taking the first step towards a more fulfilling and pleasurable sex life! By reading this book, you have gained valuable insights and tips on how to increase vaginal lubrication, get aroused faster, and overcome painful intercourse.

A. Recap of Key Points from the Book

Throughout this book, we have discussed a variety of techniques and strategies for improving vaginal lubrication, including:

- Natural remedies such as eating a healthy diet, staying hydrated, and performing Kegel exercises
- Using lubricants and moisturizers to increase lubrication and reduce discomfort during sex

Cheryl Bach

- Exploring different forms of stimulation, such as clitoral stimulation and nipple play
- Engaging in foreplay and setting the mood with lighting, music, and sensual touches
- Communicating openly with your partner about your needs and desires

We have also touched on the importance of taking care of your sexual health, including the need for regular gynecological appointments, tracking your menstrual cycle, and practicing safe sex.

B. Encouragement to Explore and Experiment with Different Techniques

It's important to remember that everyone's body and experience with sexuality are unique. While some techniques mentioned in this book may work for you, others may not. It's important to explore and experiment with different techniques to find what works best for you and your partner.

Don't be afraid to try new things or step outside of your comfort zone. By being open to new experiences and communicating openly with your partner, you can discover new levels of pleasure and satisfaction.

C. Empowerment for the Reader to Take Care of their Sexual Health and Pleasure

Ultimately, the goal of this book is to empower you to take control of your sexual health and pleasure. By understanding your body and exploring what works for you, you can break through any dry spells and experience more pleasure and intimacy in your sex life.

Remember to prioritize communication, both with yourself and your partner, and to seek out medical help if you are experiencing any pain or discomfort during intercourse.

Cheryl Bach

Above all, don't be afraid to embrace your sexuality and take pleasure in your body and desires. You deserve to feel fulfilled and satisfied in your sexual experiences, and by following the tips and techniques outlined in this book, you can achieve just that.

Thank you for reading "How to Get Wet for Sex: 25+ Hot and Slippery Ways to Increase Vaginal Lubrication, Get Aroused Really Fast, and Break Your Dry Spell plus Tips to Solve Vaginal Dryness and Overcome Painful Intercourse" - we hope it has helped you on your journey towards a happier, healthier, and more satisfying sex life. Always remember to prioritize your pleasure, communicate openly, and explore what works for you. By doing so, you can experience the joys and benefits of a fulfilling and vibrant sexual relationship.

We wish you the best of luck in all your future sexual endeavors, and we're confident that with the knowledge and techniques outlined in this book, you'll be able to achieve the fulfilling and pleasurable sex life you've always dreamed of.

Thank you once again for reading, and we hope that this book has been both informative and enjoyable for you!

Cheryl Bach

www.ingramcontent.com/pod-product-compliance
Lightning Source LLC
Chambersburg PA
CBHW051716250726
48653CB00007B/3065